Happy as a Clam, Sick as a Dog or Dead as a Doornail?

Using the "Human Life Cycle" approach for chronic disease prevention
and a longer, healthier life.

By Michael S. Weislik

Marek Ventures LLC

Oak Park, California

Happy as a Clam, Sick as a Dog or Dead as a Doornail?

Published by Marek Ventures LLC, 653 Oak Run Trail, Oak Park, CA 91377

Cover and book design by Mike Weislik.

Photographs used with permission and licenses from Fotolia.com.

ISBN-13: 978-09837618-0-8

Printed in the United States.

First printing- August 2011.

Library of Congress Control Number: 2011913796

AN IMPORTANT NOTE: This book is offered for informational purposes only and is protected by freedom of speech. It is not intended as a substitute for the medical recommendations of physicians or other health care providers. Rather, it is intended to offer information to help the reader cooperate with physicians and health professionals in a mutual quest for optimum well being. Always work with your qualified health professionals before making any changes to your diet, prescription drug use, lifestyle or exercise activities. This information is provided as is and the publisher and author expressly disclaim all liability, as the reader assumes all risk from its use, non-use or misuse of this information.

DEDICATION:

To my father, who could have lived a longer life cycle had he been more aware of the un-holistically designed systems, culture and products of the industrial revolution and made more preventative, precautionary and sustainable choices.

Happy as a Clam, Sick as a Dog or Dead as a Doornail?

TABLE OF CONTENTS

INTRODUCTION

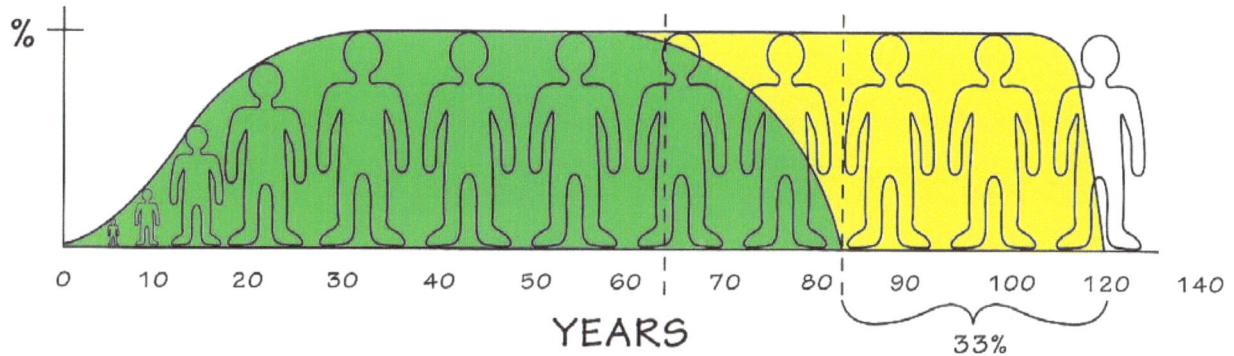

How's your human life cycle doing? In the next hour or so I'd like to talk to you about that life cycle and what maybe shortening it prematurely and some tasks you can do to lengthen your potential human life cycle activity potential. As a systems thinker, I will synthesize my thoughts and those of many other thought leaders on health, so you can benefit from this collective intelligence, wisdom and merging of strategies that together will produce a result that individually each piece does not. Please take a moment now to mark this page so you can return to it, and take a look at the references at the end of this book. I know this may seen unusual, but please check out the references.

These are the thought leaders I've chosen to help frame this story. Once you're done, come back and we'll get started again.

Happy as a Clam, Sick as a Dog or Dead as a Doornail?

What does it take to live to be 100 years old or more? Why is it that some folks live longer than others and others die prematurely? Where do sayings like, "sick as a dog", "dead as a doornail" or "happy as a clam" come from anyway? And how are these related?

It seems like the answers to these questions should be either very easy or very complex. It's actually both, in my opinion. In both cases, it's more of a journey rather than a destination. We've got human culture and your human body. Your human body is very resilient in terms of survival, but there are limits. We'll see how these limits are created and how you can extend these limits and potentially live a longer life. In terms of changing your life, it doesn't necessitate a new "start from day one approach". But the sooner you start the better the prevention against a whole host of potential health issues. Like the sayings, "sick as a dog", "dead as a door nail" or "happy as a clam", our culture develops common phrases over time to describe our conditions and approaches to life's many activities, including our approach to health and old age.   For most folks, our goal might be "happy as a clam, at high tide" (a phrase that clam diggers use, for the fortunate clams that stay protected and live longer, since the high tide keeps diggers away). Let's see how you can create your high tide and protect yourself, since no one wants to be "sick as a dog", or "dead as a doornail", at least not prematurely.

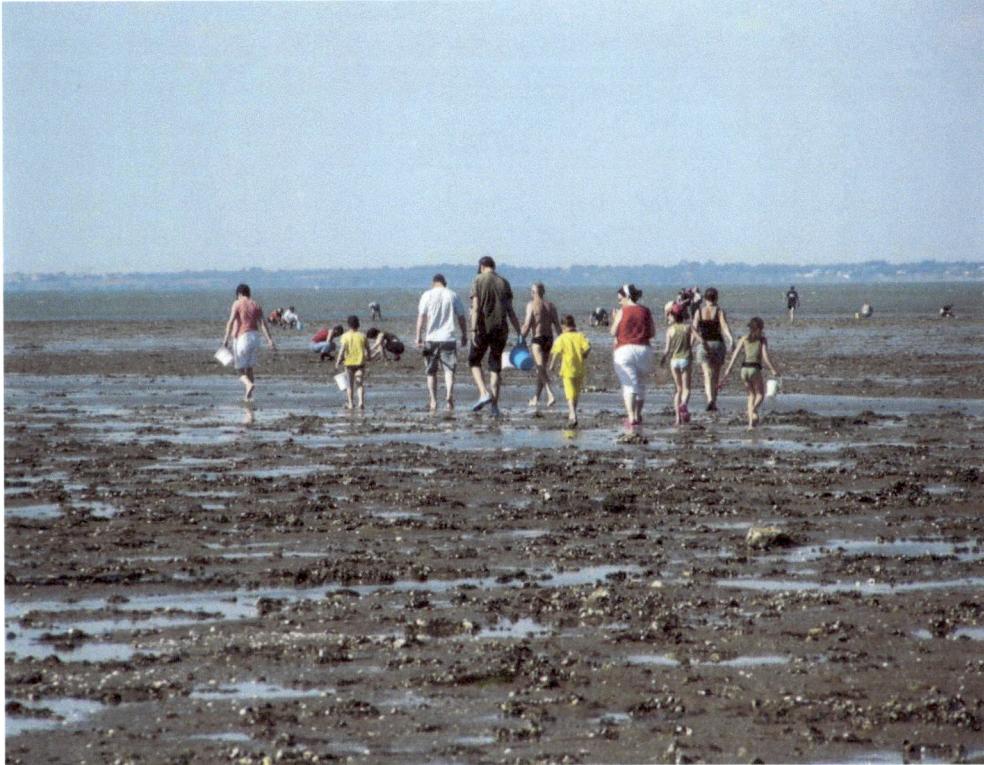

PART 1
Systems and Bathtubs

Happy as a Clam, Sick as a Dog or Dead as a Doornail?

The process starts with awareness, and understanding that you are part of a "system". Systems are groups of interacting elements that make up a complex whole. So the first question we should ask is, what kind of "system" are we looking at?

Systems can be modeled, and one classic model is of stocks. flows and feedback loops. . This is best represented as a bath tub[1]. The stock is the water level in the tub, the flows are the input water faucet and output drain, and the feedback loop is the control of the rate of which the water flows in, versus out of the tub.   Stocks, like the water in the tub, are like the amount of impurities you ingest in your body, or the amount of sugar (glycemic load), protein, fat, salt or potassium, among many others, that you put in your body, or your tub. Stocks take time to change, because flows take time to flow. Stocks act like delays or buffers or shock absorbers in systems, and are the memory of the history of changing flows within a system.

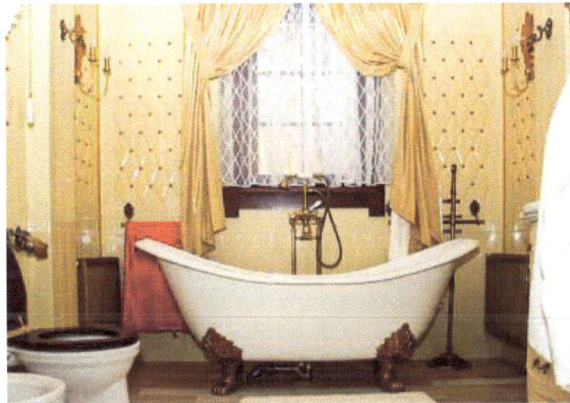

The bathtub model gives you an idea that maybe there is a limit to how much your body can do, based on the amount of intakes or flows you subject your body to. Too much input with out enough output to your body, and like the tub, it overflows.

These overflows or imbalances cause disease. It should be clearer now to see that redefining our choices and understanding their impacts can prevent disease and prolong healthy life. An example of this is your midsection. This is one of many feedback indicators of your body's health. High glycemic loads over time will give you increased insulin resistance and excessive fat reserves in your midsection. Of course, it maybe difficult to resist indulgences, since many of us have a mental model of consumption and hedonistic virtue, bestowed upon us by our culture. This consumption bathtub is one that exists in our minds, with a strong re-enforcing feedback loop. Self indulgence leads to more happiness, but worse health, which leads to even more indulgence, and even worse health until the cycle brings an overflow to your body. Your indulgence is the increased rate of flow into your tub, the water level your happiness, the decreased output drain your decreased state of health, and the overflow, disease, collapse or death. Another bathtub could be your stress levels. Inputs that come from traffic or problems at work, build up like the water in your tub, but with exercise or meditation, you can open and increase the flow of the drain to relieve the stress from your body. This is akin to toxins, since they too also build up in our bodies, and need to be drained out, thru detoxification practices.

If you do not recognize these tubs and feedback loops that keep your body healthy, you will experience disease.

Your body seeks resonance, so it constantly works to try to rebalance what it can, but it cannot always do so without your help and awareness. Like the chords of music we hear, these balances of stocks are harmonious to our overall health, but you must learn how to put these notes together in resonance again, to be healthier. The parable of the boiled frog[2] teaches us about this awareness. Put a frog in a pot of cool water and it will just sit there. Put the frog in a pot of hot water and it will jump out immediately. But put a frog in a pot of cool water, and then slowly turn up the temperature of the water, and the frog will remain in the pot and grow groggier and groggier and eventually will die. Why is that? The frog's internal apparatus for sensing threats to survival is geared toward sudden changes in the environment, not slow, gradual changes. This is like the bathtubs or stocks in our bodies. And why one day you might wake up and have a heart attack or discover you have cancer? Where was the warning sign? You won't get one, until an over flow. Some overflows take only a few days, others maybe a few years. Understanding the systems we live in helps us find and avoid over flows and bring the resonance we need for balanced bodily stocks.

The additional benefit of balanced body systems is resilience…the ability to recover from perturbation or the ability to restore or repair itself.

Systems thinking is a discipline for seeing the "structures" that underlie complex situations, and for discerning high from low leverage change. System structure is the source of system behavior[3]. In addition to bath tubs, there is another structure or archetype called "shifting the burden to the intervener"[4]. This structure can be defined as a symptomatic solution that temporarily alleviates a problem symptom, but it disconnects the signal to invest in a more fundamental solution and creates side effects that further divert attention away from a fundamental solution. A good example of this archetype is when certain doctors tell us very little on how to stay healthy and care for us only upon urgent, critical care request, so we don't pay very much attention to our nutrition, which fundamentally determines how our bodies will create our true long term health.

Hopefully by now, you've started to see the systems that are a part of you and have stepped outside of them, to see the bigger systems that are driving them. If not, it will happen soon, as you reflect on these words, the next chapter, and seek deeper answers to questions you have about your health.

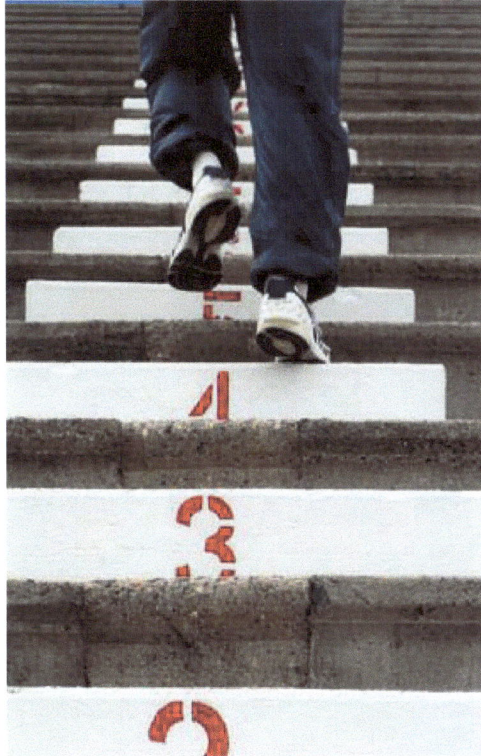

PART 2
Human Life Cycle Steps

Happy as a Clam, Sick as a Dog or Dead as a Doornail?

Happy as a Clam, Sick as a Dog or Dead as a Doornail?

What's a bigger system? Let's call this one the Economic system. We're all familiar with our 9-5, day to day, with our got to go to work mindset, so we can live fast, die young and leave a good looking corpse, right? (Another phrase from American culture.)

It's easy to be too busy with your job or family to keep track of your health, really. You might say, "that's what I have a health plan and a doctor for, right? You might never really notice any long term side effects of the lifestyle you've chosen, because, in many ways, you don't feel the consequences of it. You may not even see it.

You might say, "The goal is what feels good and gives me pleasure, right?"

Well when you're in the economic system, it's like walking up a great big, steep, hill. You never get to look up much because you're looking where you're stepping and the hill is always smack dab in front of you. When you reach the top, or your supposed retirement phase of your life, you're lucky if your health will support you for a few years, let alone 20 or maybe 50+ more years, since for the most part, you've burned yourself out getting to the top. But it's at the top where we see the big picture, isn't it? We can finally see where we've been and where we're going.

But you say, "I'm working out, and try to keep fit, so I should be OK, right?" But a better question to ask is, are you really healthy on the inside, in each organ, tissue and cell?

Does your doctor check that? "Not really at that level, unless there's a problem, usually."

But, are you aware that a majority of chronic diseases are caused by accumulations of extended exposures, environmental toxins[5] and food additives over long periods of time?

"What's that?"

Sure, if you're putting stuff in your body that your body has never been exposed to before or over exposed to and doesn't know what to do with, it stores them somewhere if the immune system can't get rid of it. Usually, it's in the tissues, organs and intercellular spaces.

"OK, so what can I do to stop the accumulations or limit these exposures?"

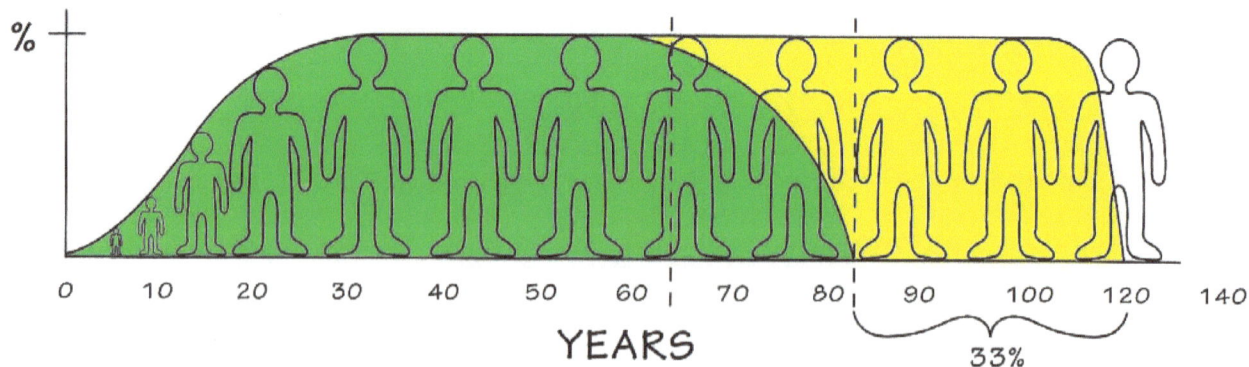

Happy as a Clam, Sick as a Dog or Dead as a Doornail?

It is time to talk about centenarians. If you are not familiar with the term, centenarians are humans that live past 100 years of age. Today, if you live in the United States, your relative life cycle activity potential starts to drop off around retirement age, and by then, you may have already had coronary by-pass surgery and/or have been diagnosed with diabetes. Your bodily systems may have been in decline for many years. The human life cycle is ~122 years, so even if you limp along and die at 82, you've lost 33% of your human life cycle relative to 122 years, or 50% of your demonstrated life cycle, relative to your 82 years. Think about those numbers for awhile. Are you losing 33% or more of your human lifecycle or HLC? That's not a really good return on your investment. The good news is that there are ways to improve this, stop accumulations and limit your exposures. Let's take a closer look at the HLC (Human Life Cycle) Steps.

HLC Step 1:

Awareness

Start treating your body like a temple. In order to do that, you've got to think outside the system, or the economy. A lot of the foods that we are tempted to buy at supermarkets and eat at many restaurants, are aimed at pleasure, convenience, or both and not at your "long term" health.

It's something called pre-meditated ignorance or sentiment abuse. It seems there are many capitalists who either do understand the consequences of their actions and don't care, or do care, but don't want to get caught, or don't understand the consequences at all or basically don't care either way, as long as the consumers are buying the product and/or service. Yes, it's OK to make money, but are you, the consumer, paying for more than you think?

It's good to note here that there is a lot of great food out there to eat, but the big question is how to know the good stuff, from the bad stuff. How do you make better choices that over a life time would give you, a human being, the potential to live a longer life (and be a happy clam, at high tide?) It's important to know here, that you are making the choices that affect your life. Take control, and be cautious of letting someone else make these decisions for you.

Happy as a Clam, Sick as a Dog or Dead as a Doornail?

When you look at the cultures around the world where individuals live well past 100 years of age, one of a few basic overall observations becomes apparent. There are no processed foods. Meaning no chemically derived additives, sweeteners, preservatives, antibiotics, pesticides, herbicides, plastics, etc.). Food preparation is daily, fresh, local and clean (organic). If food is preserved, it is done through drying and some salting (where salt is available). It's a very basic concept.....If nature didn't create it on nature's terms, then they don't eat it.

Where we're going here is to really understand more deeply, the science of true health, i.e. our food. Everything you put into your body has an effect on your body, so it makes some sense that if we take a closer look at our food and eating habits, we may find out some ways to get cleaner running fuel for a longer life.

Bottom Line: Recognize that the system you're in, does not always have your best interest in mind, in terms of your long term health.

HLC Step 2:

Eliminate Contamination/Alterations in all Primary Body inputs from environmental exposures.

A) Air: Avoid smoking, inhaling diesel fumes, or any other air borne toxins that maybe in your environment. You have to become more aware of your environment to do this, so walk around in your home, office and living spaces to see what's out there. A lesser known air borne toxin is clothes dryer vent exhaust that comes from the perfume laced chemicals used in certain fabric softener products, dryer sheets, and many detergents. If your laundry products are not based on 100% natural ingredients, why would you want to wear clothes that are washed and dried that have chemicals that your skin will absorb, and over time, create degenerative disease?

B) Water: drink distilled, reverse osmosis or filtered water. Avoid plastic bottled water and plasticizers[6], by replacing or using your own glass or stainless steel containers. Distilled water is preferred since that is what you eat when you have a piece of fruit[7]. Nature has done the filtering for you, in this case.

C) Food: Eat your own home grown vegetables, organic and GMO free food. The USDA Organic label indicates 95% organic ingredients, or 5% potential non-organic ingredients and you can select 100% organic, it that is indicated as well. Of course, local farmer's markets or organic farm shopping makes sense if you're not growing your own. Your next best option is organic frozen and last choice is canned.

D) Drugs: Limit your use of prescription drugs. If you've already in a chronic health situation, then its best to review each drug carefully with your doctor to ensure that it is an absolute, life or death situation that requires it. Keep in mind there are strong political and economic reasons for doctors and drug companies to sell prescription drugs, other than to try to improve a health issue. On the other hand, the human body is an amazing self-healing system, provided you give your body enough time and the "natural" inputs to make the healing possible. Many prescription drugs only mask health issues or acute symptoms and can have long term consequences that have not been determined yet, even though they maybe FDA approved. Remember that the right food can improve health issues and serve your body's own immune system.

Bottom Line: Start really looking at what you've putting in your body. What you breathe in, eat, drink, and what touches your skin, all have an effect on your health, especially your long term health.

HLC Step 3:

Re-balance fat, salt and sugar inputs and understand their relation to your body's PH.

Each year for the last 40 years, the average amount of fat, salt and sugar has increased in processed foods. Many processed foods in most American supermarkets are becoming more like candy every day. Why? Generally speaking it's about retaining you as a customer. The strategy is to get you hooked on the product so you'll buy more, and residual corporate incomes can be established. So for food, adding more salt, sugar and/or fat works, since this appeals to your sensory glands, your urge to add more pleasure to your life and again, makes many foods taste like candy.

Once your body gets accustomed to this cycle, your urges to continue maybe addictive. Its great to have a treat once in awhile, but this is where the system is not working for your long term best interest.

For example, many marinated meats are loaded with sugar and salt, not to mention many frozen vegetables loaded with butter (fat, salt, sugar). Countless canned products use salt as a preservative, but add excessive amounts of salt (sodium) to add extra zest and appeal to the recipe. Excessive daily sodium (salt) intake can raise blood pressure. Note that a considerable amount is in processed foods. You must read nutrition labels to ascertain your daily/weekly intake levels. If you don't, you'll probably end up a victim of this process (and your bathtub will overflow).

As for fats, start first by avoiding all foods that contain trans fats (hydrogenated oils). Then reduce your consumption of saturated fats. One of my favorite examples on this topic is grain fed meats. For thousands of years before the industrial revolution, domesticated animals grazed in fields on grasses. Then during the course of the industrialization of animal production, the discovery of grain feeding produced a mature cow for market in half the time of a grass fed cow, and a new way to speed up the production/profit cycle began. This process also added additional marbling that added more saturated fat, and more flavorful meat (remember, from a fat perspective, fat is stored sugar). What also changed, but is not widely talked about, are the EFA Omega 6/Omega 3 fatty acid profiles of the meat. Grass fed meats are about ~1:1. whereas grain fed meats are ~30:1. EFA's are essential fatty acids and the ones the body needs, but cannot make on its own. They are used by every living cell in the body, and the 30:1 imbalance impedes the body's ability to suppress inflammation/ infection and build new cells properly. Which means you're weakening an essential component of your immune system by eating grain-fed meats. Note also that Omega 3 EFAs are also a vital component of brain tissue. At any age, an imbalance of EFA Omega 6/ Omega 3 will cause issues with the cognitive functions of the brain, and limit the proper maintenance of cells in the brain. Many researchers today feel this is the cause of diseases like attention deficit hyperactive disorder (ADHD) and depression, to name a few. The key here is to reduce Omega 6 intakes and increase Omega 3 intakes and obtain balance. How do you do this? If you eat red meat, by buy organic, grass fed meats or game meats and/or start using Omega 3 oils like flaxseed oil, as a supplement. This will reduce your saturated fat intake, and increase beneficial oils in your body. Remember that flaxseed oil is not for cooking, so just add it to your salads or vegetable dishes as a dressing. Use olive oil for your cooking purposes.

It is hard to find any processed food product today that doesn't have high fructose corn syrup as an ingredient. This overwhelming pervasiveness has lead many people to have very high glycemic loads, or day to day glycemic levels that are very high. This can also be described as very high carbohydrate load. This loading is a primary component for developing insulin resistance[8], increased obesity and the diabetes epidemic. Some of the primary culprits here are table sugar, foods made with high fructose corn syrup (HFCS) and/or refined grains, like white flour. These are foods that you should try to eliminate completely in your diet.

Let's look at high fructose corn syrup. HFCS was developed by a soft drink company's research laboratory[9] as a low cost substitute for cane sugar. After its introduction, this company was able to utilize the increased margins and profits to buy back control of its independent bottlers to increase its end product pricing, and ultimately increase its market capitalization. HFCS has been pervasive in the food processing industry ever since, in terms of its wider channel penetration and consumer reach. The effects on human health have not been as cheery, since this ingredient is now helping to turn most processed food that contain it into candy. Yes, there are many manufacturers that do not use HFCS, but you'll need to keep checking labels and shop in some other stores to find these brands..

Your body is continually trying to balance its pH. When this balance is compromised many problems can occur. Over exposures to excessive amounts of sugar, salt and bad fats create this imbalance. Get some litmus paper and check your saliva and urine. The best time to check is one hour before or two hours after a meal. On the 0-14 scale, normal human saliva is 6.5-7.5 through out the day, and urine 6.0-6.5 in the morning and 6.5-7.0 in the evening. In order to sustain these levels, your diet should come from 80% alkaline forming foods and 20% acid forming foods. In general, animal products are acid producing and vegetable are alkaline forming. Its is best of go online and look at the many charts available to see the most acidic and most alkaline foods, so you can keep your diet in balance. It's easy, just look-up "food pH".

Bottom Line: Get more omega 3 fats into your diet by replacing omega 6's with flax seed oils or another omega 3 fat source that works for you. Lower sodium and increase potassium intakes. Reduce your daily glycemic loads by reducing or eliminating your intake of table sugar, processed sugars like HFCS, or white flour. Monitor your body pH. The additional wisdom here is that by using your blood type, you can determine where your best sources of proteins, carbohydrates and various fats should come from and we'll cover this in the next section.

HLC Step 4:

Review Compatibility

Why is it that the human species has different blood types? Think about this from another perspective. Our ancient ancestors generally lived in isolated areas, consuming a limited variety of foods, indigenous to that area. As they moved into new areas over thousands of years, blood types changed through evolution to deal with new food sources, infections and disease. But today, with the modern supermarket, there is so much worldly variety, how is it that our bodies can be compatible to all foods? The answer is very simple. We cannot be, since we are genetically pre-dispositioned by blood types. Your blood type influences every area of your physiology on a cellular level. It has every thing to do with how your digest your food, your ability to respond to stress, your mental state, the efficiency of your metabolism, and the strength of your immune system.. Its really common sense that certain foods would be highly beneficial to the human body and others would act like poisons based on your blood type[10]. There is a lot of great research and books on this subject by Dr. Peter D'Adamo, and it's very important to gain an understanding of the importance of accumulated lectin damage, and the relationship it has to the health of your immune system. Additionally, genes do not determine disease on their own. Genes function only by being activated, or expressed, and nutrition plays a critical role in determining which genes, good or bad, are expressed.[11]

Bottom Line: Determine your blood type and review the blood type charts on beneficial/non-beneficial foods and focus on selecting more beneficial foods for your body. Through your diet choices, you'll avoid lectin damage and start expressing your good genes and repressing your bad genes that are inherently part of your blood type, family and human heritage.

HLC Step 5:

Exercise/Skeletal Movement/Sleep

Humans were designed for exercise, so get out and do something that gives you some movement and preferably some sweating. Sweating is evidence of aerobic activity for your body. Some of the American culture is a bit extremist based, so running 5K, 10K or Iron Man/Woman competitions are OK if you're motivated to do so, but this level of aerobic activity, in my opinion, is not needed for long term health. Some folks will disagree, but oxidation is a primary ingredient for cellular aging, in connection with protein production processes in our bodies. Over-exercising means over-oxidation. Again, in my opinion, go for moderation in exercise. In addition to the "sweating" exercise, humans should include a minimum level of skeletal/muscular resistance in this routine to maintain the strength of joints, tendons and connective tissues that keep the body from getting routine aches and pains. Also, exercise helps the human pituitary gland to produce HGH. Human growth hormone is a chemical signal that keeps your body systems in repair.

A great way to increase activity in your lifestyle is to own a pet. Dogs are great since they need to be walked twice a day to stay healthy, and this helps the owner get into the habit of exercising as well. Putting your dog on a running line is not preferred, since you'll lose the exercise benefit, as well as the mutual bonding time with your dog.

As for sleep, this is the time of day when your body does its repairs, so getting a full 8 hours is very important. Some folks think that as they get older they need less sleep, but this is because your body has slowed down its repair cycle. This is a sign that your body is aging. If you exercise more, your need for sleep will increase and it may add more years to your life, as a positive consequence.

Bottom Line: Get daily exercise, enough so you sleep 8 hours. This is a way to gauge your exercise commitment level. Remember that exercise helps your lymphatic system to move waste fluids from your systems for proper elimination.

HLC Step 6:

Vitamins and Minerals

Most of industrialized society is a victim of not having sufficient vitamins and minerals in our bodies. The idea of heat-processing food, in most cases, neutralizes most natural forms of vitamins and reduces mineral impacts. Why do you think cereal boxes display the vitamins and minerals they have? The manufacturers have to add these losses back in to the product help market the products with some health benefits. Eating organic and raw foods gives the best form, quality and quantity of vitamins and minerals, since these are foods crafted by nature, not a manufacturing process. Imbalances in your vitamins and minerals can cause a whole host of issues for your health. Naturopathic practitioners like Dr. Weil, generally recommend at least some basic supplementation[12] to make up for losses created by the processed food manufacturers and modern agriculture. These include selenium, vitamin C, vitamin E, mixed carotenoids, B-complex vitamin, calcium as well as

vitamin D if you are not getting ~15-20 minutes of sunlight per day.

Bottom Line: Start eating your own garden vegetables, buy organic vegetables and fruits and take a

daily supplement of vitamins and minerals to make up for imbalances in your body's systems.

HLC Step 7:

Antioxidants

With all of today's modern industrial activities, our bodies face an overwhelming amount of

toxins that in many cases, we are not even aware of. After reviewing Dr. Packer's work at

Berkeley[13], it is evident that are bodies are not equipped to take on this battle without help, or we face

potential accelerated aging. His basic antioxidant recommendations are similar to Dr. Weil's except

that he adds in boosting glutathione levels as an additional anti-aging antioxidant. This is best done

by eating foods like spinach and/or supplementing with lipoic acid.[14]

Bottom Line: If you're eating lots of garden vegetables and organic fruits and vegetables and you are taking some vitamin and mineral supplements, you're on the right track to getting daily antioxidants, so consider more spinach and also supplementing with lipoic acid.

HLC Step 8:

Absorption

Why is it that the human species is the only species that cooks its food? Well, most folks would say that cooked food tastes better. But in the process of cooking, did the food change from its natural state? Yes, it lost most of its enzymes[15]. Even though our pancreas produces enzymes, with overwhelming amounts of cooked food, the pancreas is in overdrive most of the time. If that is the case, then what other functions might the pancreas not be doing as much of to make up for the extra capacity for enzyme production?   The point I'm trying to make is that eating food as close to its natural, organic state is best. Not required, but best, since most of the enzymes stay intact. Enzymes are the precursors to thousands of metabolic processes, so any shortage of these, just prevents other things from happening. There's just a lot more to food than fat, protein and carbs.

Bottom Line: If you're still eating a lot of cooked food, consider supplementing with daily enzymes, to give your pancreas and your immune system a boost..

HLC Step 9:

Combining

Its basic chemistry that if you mix acid and base foods, you're going to get a reaction, usually gas, cramps, etc. Although this step remains very subjective, I believe it's good to try to follow your body's rhythms and recognize that combinations of foods can create problems for your body, and have a potential long term effect on your body. Harvey and Marilyn Diamond make a strong case for this approach as part of Natural Hygiene for a healthy lifestyle[16].

Bottom Line: If there are food combinations that give you gas, recognize this and try to avoid combining these foods to avoid other non-beneficial side effects as well.

HLC Step 10:

Sequencing

It's always fascinating that if you get a small cut during the day, how after you sleep that night, the cut is already healed a bit. When you think about this for awhile you might get the sense that there is a cycle or rhythm to our bodies, like active during the day, and inactive at night. Even though our bodies are constantly re-building, our rest periods intensify the re-building process during our "physically" in-active state. This brings up the importance of rest, and especially sleep when you body is telling you to. The more and better quality sleep, the better the re-building. As for food, it only makes sense that since the body has been re-building during sleep, that by the morning, food is needed for your brain and cells. The faster your breakfast metabolizes the better, since it will get into your cells and help wake you up. Remember, breakfast means "breaking from fasting all night". The foods that metabolize the fastest are fruits and juices.

Bottom Line: Follow your body's pattern of intake and absorption, assimilation and elimination by starting your day with lighter foods like fruits and juices, then progress to heavier foods as the day moves on, and stop eating by mid evening.

HLC Step 11:

Colon and Heavy Metal Detox

This is where you can give your body another way to rest a bit, and at the same time, give your body a way to remove toxin build up in muscles, fat reserves and organs. Colon detox allows your immune system to get revved up and do some "cleaning" work that it may not be able to do during "normal or regular" food intake patterns[17]. Again from environmental exposures our bodies can accumulate excessive amounts of heavy metals that should be monitored just like your standard blood tests, normally once per year. There are hair and fecal matter versions of this test and can provide insight into where to focus your detox efforts. Harvey Diamond has another version of this he calls periodic"monodieting"[18].

Bottom Line: Plan to do a preliminary detox of your systems followed by an annual detox routine. You can always add more detoxes during the year, but its based on your lifestyle and dietary habits. This helps to keep your bathtubs clean, too.

HLC Step 12:

Mind Body Awareness

Begin to practice daily meditation or any relaxation response to keep your stress levels in check[19]. This includes activities like yoga or tai chi for inner chi development.

Spend time outside in Nature to purify your senses and bring them back to their source in nature.

Also nurture positive and secure relationships that are life-supporting[20].

Bottom Line: There will always be a connection between your mind, your body and your health.

Keeping your senses and reactions in tune with what your body is telling you. This helps to keep you healthy. Calming your mind will help you to cleanse your mind as well.

Happy as a Clam, Sick as a Dog or Dead as a Doornail?

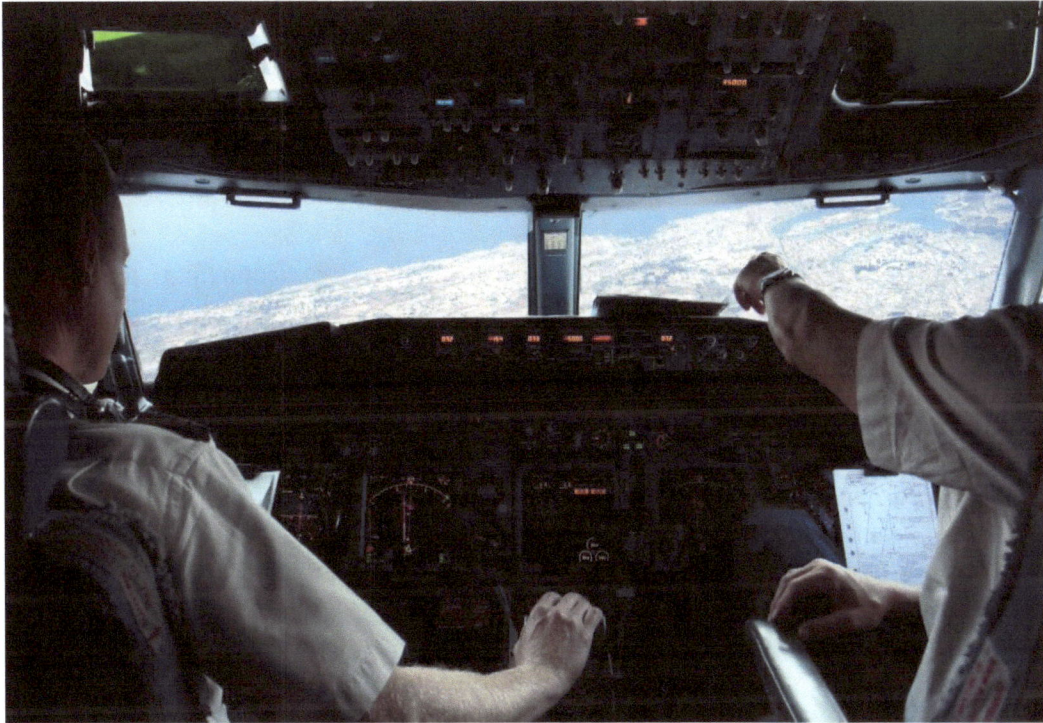

CONCLUSION

Our economic/health system is not an intrinsically responsible system today since the system does

not send feedback about the consequences of a decision directly, quickly and compellingly to the decision maker. An example of an intrinsic system is an airplane and its pilot. Because the pilot of a plane rides in front of the plane, he or she is intrinsically responsible, since he or she will experience directly the consequences of his or her decisions. With this plane analogy in mind, a few doctors are moving from the back of the plane to the front, since they are taking an interest in your flight to long-term health. Dr. Packer, Rogers, Schwarzbein, D'Adamo, Clapp, Weil and Chopra, among others, have become mentors and guiding counsel for long term health. The existing economic food system will take years out of your lifecycle, unless you make some changes, take control, and put your life on a path to a healthier approach. Nature designs incredible foods yet our system is filled with many poorly designed processed foods for pleasure and profit. Dr. Campbell states that the system promotes profit over health, technology over food and confusion over clarity[21]. Additionally, he adds that nutrition training of doctors is not merely inadequate, it is practically non-existent[22]. With that in mind, here is a summary of a healthier systematic approach, one that can potentially extend your lifecycle and allow you to be a healthy, happier clam, and maybe a centenarian.

Remember to maximize the whole, and not just a few parts. Sub-optimization is less effective as a strategy. Focus on enhancing properties of the whole, and keeping your stocks in balance, thus eliminating toxic accumulations/and overflows. Open a dialog with your doctor about all dietary and lifestyle changes.

HLC STEP SUMMARY

- Recognize that the economic system you're in does not always have your best interest in mind, in terms of your long term health.

- Start really looking at what you've putting in and on your body. What you breathe in, eat, drink, and what touches your skin all have an effect on your health, especially your long term health.

- Drink clean water, breathe in clean, fresh air, and avoid all unnecessary toxic exposures. This means re-thinking the products you choose to use on a daily basis during your daily activities, as well as some of your activity choices. Do you understand the impacts of the chemicals you're exposing your body to? Are you aware that these chemicals exist?

- Reduce your daily glycemic loads by reducing or eliminating your intake of table sugar, processed sugars, like HFCS, or white flour products. Monitor your body pH. The goal is 80% alkaline forming foods and 20% acid forming foods and you'll be in the normal pH ranges. Use the internet and look up "food pH".

- Get more omega 3 fats into your diet by replacing omega 6's. Some suggestions are flax seed oil (as a dressing), and/or eating grass fed meats. Lower your sodium and increase your potassium intakes. The additional wisdom here is that by using your blood type, you can determine where your better sources of proteins, carbohydrates and various fats should come from.

- Determine your blood type, look up and review the charts on beneficial/non-beneficial foods and focus on selecting more beneficial foods for your body. Through your diet choices, you'll be expressing your good genes and repressing your bad genes that are inherently part of your blood type, family and human heritage.

- Get daily exercise, enough so you sleep 8 hours. This is a way to gauge your exercise commitment level. Remember that exercise helps your lymphatic system to move waste

- fluids from your systems for proper elimination. Seldom talked about but a critical component to your long term health.

- Start eating your own garden vegetables, and/or buy organic vegetables and fruits plus consider taking a daily supplement of vitamins and minerals to make up for imbalances in your body's systems.

- If you're eating lots of garden or organic vegetables and fruits plus you are taking some vitamin and mineral supplements, you're on the right track to getting your daily antioxidant intakes, so also consider eating more spinach and/or supplementing with lipoic acid for even longer term benefits.

- If you're still eating a lot of cooked food, consider supplementing with daily enzymes, to give your pancreas a rest and your immune system a boost.

- If there are food combinations that give you gas, recognize this and try to avoid combining these foods to avoid other non-beneficial side effects as well.

- Follow your body's pattern of intake and absorption, assimilation and elimination by starting your day with lighter foods like fruits and juices, then progress to heavier foods as the day moves on. Stop eating by mid evening.

- Plan to do a preliminary detoxification of your body systems followed by an annual detoxification routine. You can always add more detoxes during the year, but their frequency is based on your lifestyle and dietary habits.

- There will always be a connection between your mind, your body and your health. Keeping your senses and reactions in tune with what your body is telling you. This helps to keep you healthy. Calming your mind will help you to cleanse your mind as well. Consider starting daily meditation and/or tai chi/yoga for inner strength development.

- Relax and enjoy! You are potentially regaining 33 to 50% of your human life cycle activity potential if you remember that your choices over the long term, are what make a difference. Keep those bathtubs from overflowing. ☺

Happy as a Clam, Sick as a Dog or Dead as a Doornail?

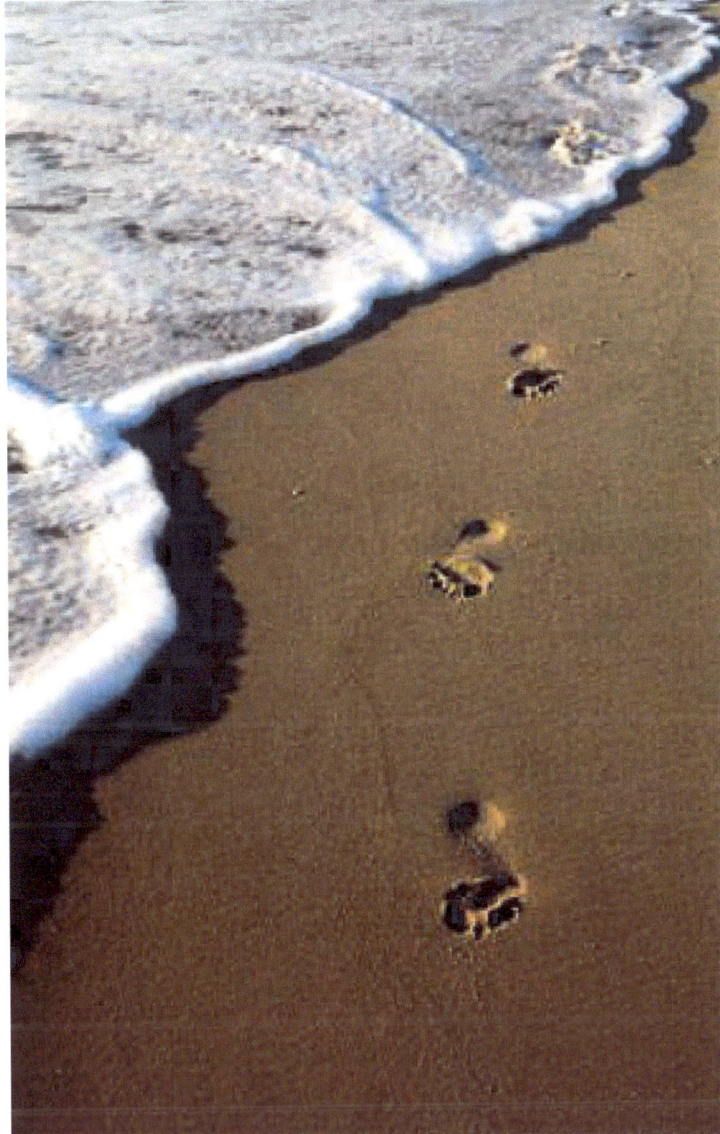

Happy as a Clam, Sick as a Dog or Dead as a Doornail?

REFERENCES

[1] Meadows, D. (2008), Thinking in Systems: *A Primer*, White River Junction: Chelsea Green Publishing. p.195.

[2] Senge, P. (1990), The Fifth Discipline: *The Art and Practice of the Learning Organization*, New York: Currency Doubleday, p.22.

[3] Meadows, D. (2008), Thinking in Systems: *A Primer*, White River Junction: Chelsea Green Publishing. p.89.

[4] Senge, P. (1990), The Fifth Discipline: *The Art and Practice of the Learning Organization*, New York: Currency Doubleday, p.382.

[5] M.D, Rogers, S. (2002), Detoxify of Die, Sarasota: Sand Key Company, p.43.

[6] ", p. 37.

[7] Diamond, H. & Diamond, M. (1985). Fit for Life, New York: MJF Books. p.44.

[8] M.D, Schwarzbein, D. (1999), The Schwarzbein Principle: The Truth about Losing Weight, Being Healthy and Feeling Younger, Dearfield Beach: Health Communications, Inc., p.8-9.

[9] Slywotsky, A. & Morrison, D. (1997), The Profit Zone: *How Strategic Business Design Will Lead You To Tomorrow's Profits,* New York: Times Books, p.144.

[10] D'Adamo, Dr. P., (1996), Eat Right For Your Type: *The Individualized Diet Solution to Staying Healthy, Living Longer & Achieving Your Ideal Weight,* New York: G.P. Putnam's Sons.

[11] Ph.D Campbell, T. & Campbell, T. (2004), The China Study: *The Most Comprehensive Study of Nutrition Ever Conducted and the Startling Implications for Diet, Weight Loss and Long-term Health*, Dallas: Benbella Books, p. 233.

[12] M.D. Weil, A. (2001), Eating Well for Optimum Health: The Essential Guide to Bringing Health and Pleasure back to Eating, New York: Quill, p. 263.

[13] Ph.D Packer, L. (1999), The Antioxidant Miracle: *Put Lipoic Acid, Pycnogenal, and Vitamins E and C to Work for You*, New York. John Wiley and Sons, Inc, p.188.

[14] ", p. 107.

[15] Diamond, H. & Diamond, M. (1985). Fit for Life, New York: MJF Books. p.42.

[16] ", p. 26.

[17] J.D., Ph.D Clapp, L. (1997), Prostate Health in 90 Days, Carlsbad: Hay House, Inc. p. 64-104.

[18] Diamond, H. (2000). Fit for Life: A New Beginning, New York: Twin Streams. p.233.

[19] J.D., Ph.D Clapp, L. (1997), Prostate Health in 90 Days, Carlsbad: Hay House, Inc. p. 226.

[20] M.D. Chopra, D. (2000), Prefect Health: The Complete Mind Body Guide, New York: Three Rivers Press, p. 241.

[21] Ph.D Campbell, T. & Campbell, T. (2004), The China Study: *The Most Comprehensive Study of Nutrition Ever Conducted and the Startling Implications for Diet, Weight Loss and Long-term Health*, Dallas: Benbella Books, p. 250.

[22] ", p. 327

ABOUT THE AUTHOR:

A graduate student integrating sustainable business practices, systems thinking, system dynamics and industrial ecology for the optimal well-being for all species. My background begins with 25 years in research and development, manufacturing, operations and global supply chain management, and provides ample acumen of how products and services have made it into our lives and into the systems that create our current health and well-being.

.

www.ingramcontent.com/pod-product-compliance
Lightning Source LLC
Chambersburg PA
CBHW060831270326
41933CB00002B/49